The College of Occupational Therapists' Curriculum Guidance for Pre-registration Education

Revised edition

College of Occupational Therapists

This curriculum guidance has been written primarily for educators, commissioners, practitioners, students, service users and managers.

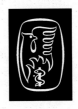

**College of
Occupational
Therapists**

Previously published in the UK in 2004 by the College of Occupational Therapists as *College of Occupational Therapists' Curriculum framework for pre-registration education*.

This edition published in 2009
by the College of Occupational Therapists
106–114 Borough High Street
London SE1 1LB
www.cot.org.uk

ISBN 978-1-905944-13-2

1/09

Typeset by Servis Filmsetting Ltd, Stockport, Cheshire
Digitally printed on demand in Great Britain by The Lavenham Press, Suffolk

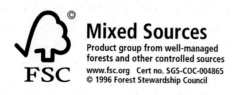

Contents

Acknowledgements   *iv*

Preface   *v*

Key terms   *vi*

Defining occupational therapy   1

The role of the College of Occupational Therapists in relation to the curriculum   2

The curriculum review process   3

Implications for the new guidance   4

A vision for occupational therapy   5

Realising the vision through education   7

The educational philosophy   9

The graduate profile   10

Appendix: Current drivers impacting on the curriculum   14

Bibliography and references   16

Acknowledgements

Thanks go to the academics, allied health professional leads, service users, private practitioners and Council of Deans representatives who participated in the Listening Event, held at the College of Occupational Therapists in March 2008, for their valuable input and advice in helping to frame this curriculum guidance.

The members of the working group that then progressed the thinking and writing and brought the guidance to fruition are also acknowledged for their expertise and commitment to the project:

Professor Auldeen Alsop

Jennifer Creek

Sally Feaver

Patricia McClure

Linda Renton

Sara Roberts

Dr Nicola Spalding

Professor Annie Turner

The College of Occupational Therapists staff that played a role in collating the output of the working group and publishing the final document are also acknowledged for their significant contribution.

This revised version of the College of Occupational Therapists' curriculum guidance is intended to inform, influence and enable the creative development of modern curricula that will lead the profession during the next decade. In setting this guidance in the context of a vision for the profession, it is anticipated that future graduates will have been exposed further to the expanding world of evidence-based occupational therapy practice in which service users play centre stage.

This guidance document intentionally allows for considerable flexibility in how university curriculum development teams address the gap between the vision and the desired outcome (the latter is expressed as a graduate profile, see pages 10–13). It is felt that this will encourage innovative and creative approaches to curriculum development.

The College expects graduates to emerge with creative and entrepreneurial capabilities as well as high-level professional and practice skills. Delivering on this expectation will enable future practitioners to be well placed in the continuing change environment of statutory health and social care. It will also enable graduates to understand and plan for their potential employment in the third sector or as independent practitioners.

This is an exciting, if challenging, time of change. Occupational therapy education needs to reflect both the excitement and the challenge through innovative and creative curricula. It will require all of those involved in the education of our future professionals – academics, practitioners, managers and placement educators – to help realise the vision and to engage with the concepts expressed within this document.

This document is offered to all those involved in the education of occupational therapists. The College entrusts you with the task of delivering its intention.

The Curriculum Review Working Group
June 2009

Key terms

This section provides an explanation of how the following terms are used within the context of this document.

Capability a dynamic concept that takes into account the skill and knowledge sufficient and suitable for a given purpose. It is characterised by the capacity for further development.

Pragmatism a philosophy that is concerned with problem-solving, activity and adaptation, and that stresses the relationship between theory and action.

Principle a general law or rule adopted or professed as a guide to action.

Professionalism implies that a person demonstrates capability in their skills and knowledge which is informed by the philosophy, values and ethical dimensions of occupational therapy practice.

Resilience the ability to deal positively and confidently with difficulties, at different periods throughout life, which challenge a person's resourcefulness and self-reliance.

Resourcefulness the ability to understand and make use of those resources (internal and external) that enable people to identify and solve problems in dynamic environments.

Self-reliance the ability to take responsibility (be autonomous) for using resources to best advantage. It is not the same as promoting independence, being independent oneself, or being independent of others.

Transformation a process of change in kind, character or nature.

Value a shared judgement of what is valuable and important in life.

Defining occupational therapy

Occupational therapists view people as occupational beings. People are intrinsically active and creative, needing to engage in a balanced range of activities in their daily lives in order to maintain health and wellbeing. People shape, and are shaped by, their experiences and interactions with their environments. They create identity and meaning through what they do and have the capacity to transform themselves through premeditated and autonomous action.

The purpose of occupational therapy is to enable people to fulfil, or to work towards fulfilling, their potential as occupational beings. Occupational therapists promote function, quality of life and the realisation of potential in people who are experiencing occupational deprivation, imbalance or alienation. They believe that activity can be an effective medium for remediating dysfunction, facilitating adaptation and recreating identity.

The role of the College of Occupational Therapists in relation to the curriculum

The College of Occupational Therapists (COT), as the professional body, has a key role to play in ensuring that pre-registration programmes in occupational therapy:

■ Reflect the current and emerging practice of occupational therapy compatible with the WFOT *Revised minimum standards for the education of occupational therapists* (Hocking and Ness 2002) and the TUNING competences for Europe (Tuning Occupational Therapy Project Group 2008) and meet the current *College of Occupational Therapists standards for pre-registration education* (COT 2008).

■ Promote the development of a dynamic occupational therapy workforce that is fit for the future.

■ Achieve the goal of supporting an evidenced-based profession committed to extending and reviewing its evidence base.

■ Enable programme teams in higher education institutions who work with practitioners, service users and students, to be creative in the development of curricula that reflect, and are responsive to, professional, political, health and social drivers.

■ Produce graduates who have comparable knowledge, capabilities and professional attributes derived from the education process.

■ Acknowledge and meet the requirements of the UK Health Professions Council (HPC) in order that graduates may apply for HPC registration.

The College, in creating this document, has set the vision for the profession and detailed the desired outcome of occupational therapy education in the form of a graduate profile. The profile is that agreed as part of the Bologna agreement to tune educational competences across Europe (Tuning Occupational Therapy Project Group 2008).

The College does not wish to prescribe the specific content of a curriculum. Instead we intend to enable the development of creative and innovative curricula that are adaptable, flexible and successful in connecting vision and outcome.

The curriculum review process

The College of Occupational Therapists produced the *curriculum framework for pre-registration education* in 2004 as a public statement of the knowledge, skills and values held by occupational therapists at the point of being eligible to apply for registration with the Health Professions Council in the United Kingdom. The *curriculum framework* represents the body of knowledge of the profession, through which the pre-registration education programmes are designed, impacting on students' subsequent employment as health professionals.

A five-year review was implemented in 2008 in keeping with the College of Occupational Therapists' standard practice for key professional documents. The review of the framework included evaluations and consultations with people across the United Kingdom, representing the interests of service users, commissioners, regulators, academics, practitioners and researchers. A working party was then set up to review the curriculum and revise the document.

In its review, the working party understood that the 2004 framework had served the profession well. It was valued for being non-prescriptive and flexible, allowing for responsive and proactive changes to take place to reflect the political and educational drivers of the day. The intent therefore was to ensure that these principles remained embedded within the revised document. The working party agreed that, in essence, the philosophy, core values and beliefs of occupational therapy remained the same. Occupation remains at the heart of the profession's practice and client-centredness leads to a people-focused curriculum. A further shift in focus from illness to wellness was needed within the new guidance, given the increasing emphasis of the various UK Governments on personal responsibility for health and the promotion of wellbeing and healthy lifestyles for all.

The key area for appraisal in the curriculum review was, however, the context of occupational therapists' employment. The new guidance would need to acknowledge the rapidly changing nature of health and social care provision and its impact on occupational therapists' practice, working lives and future development. As a result of the profession's development and focus on occupational needs, there has been a pro-active move towards establishing services in non-illness focused contexts, so broadening the range of employment opportunities for occupational therapists. There is also evidence of increasing confidence of occupational therapists in independent practice. These developments in turn impact on the curriculum, which in future must enable students to hone their leadership, business and professional skills for employability.

Implications for the new guidance

This new document has to reflect those known drivers that impact on the occupational therapy curriculum. Some flexibility is required to accommodate an anticipated and, to some extent, an unknown future for the profession. The drivers (existing and new) that were perceived to be influential in the revision of the 2004 COT framework are shown in the appendix (see pages 14–15).

The new curriculum also has to reflect the changing models of health and social care provision. It must enable graduates to recognise and articulate the role that occupation plays in the lives of service users, and ways in which occupational therapists can work for the benefit of individuals, communities and populations in emerging practice areas. In addition to professional skills, the development of personal qualities such as leadership and entrepreneurship will need to be embedded within the curriculum.

The curriculum will need to reflect current practice and influence future practice through continued innovations in academic and practice settings (including the growing use of information technology).

To this end, this new guidance will encourage and support innovation in curricula to ensure that graduate occupational therapists have future-proofed capability.

A vision for occupational therapy

For many years, occupational therapists have worked with people who have secondary and tertiary healthcare needs resulting from acute or long-term illness and disability. For the last thirty years or so, occupational therapists have been working in primary healthcare contexts to manage people's health and social care needs. Practice in these areas has reduced unnecessary admission to hospitals and care settings and has supported people in their own environments. In the past five years or so, some occupational therapists have broken new ground, working with people and communities outside of the statutory health and social care sectors, such as homeless people. The occupational therapist's role in these settings has been to enable individuals and communities to establish ways of living that are personally meaningful and sustainable. These initiatives support the achievement of people's occupational aspirations, for example as parents, employees, students or homemakers.

In all these settings, occupational therapy is a vehicle for bringing about transformation, which implies a change from one condition to another. For example, the occupational therapist attempts to engage socially disaffected people in activities and occupations that enable them to identify their own issues and needs and to work towards resolutions that have meaning for them. The approach based on this philosophy promotes the individual's personal sense of wellbeing, social engagement and participation.

In order to ensure that occupational therapy remains relevant to and valued by society, the profession itself needs to change, through:

■ **Revisiting** the power of occupation to transform lives and communities.

■ **Reimagining** the purpose of occupational therapy to create a future in which everyone is able to benefit from the transformative potential of occupation.

■ **Reconceptualising** occupational therapy intervention as a dynamic, proactive and responsive process that is a collaborative endeavour between therapist and service user.

There are three transformative processes that will support these changes:

1 **The transformation of aspects of service users' lives through engagement in occupation.**
For service users, social transformation is the process by which the right of every citizen to have equal access to, and inclusion in, services and products that sustain their health and wellbeing is upheld. The current policy drivers around personalisation bring this into even sharper focus. The occupational therapist employs a recognised process of assessment, intervention and evaluation to achieve outcomes for and with the service user. When occupation is used as a medium for transformation, the outcomes for the service user are an increase in self-reliance, resourcefulness and resilience.

2 **The transformation of students into effective practitioners.**
Transformative learning is the process through which students make the shift from novice to autonomous and effective practitioners. They come to understand the factors that support transformation, not only of themselves, but also of others,

including service users. The transformation of service users is dependent on the ability of practitioners to make a positive impact on the issues that influence health and wellbeing for individuals and communities. These issues include, for example, unemployment, homelessness, ageing populations and public health concerns such as obesity. During the process of transformation, the occupational therapist takes account of, and influences, a multitude of factors. Change in one factor may be the catalyst for other changes. The processes that occupational therapists use should thus be viewed as dynamic and complex, yet unrestrictive in guiding problem solving and decision-making.

3 **The transformation of the profession in response to changing contexts of service delivery.**
There have been recent changes to the shape and organisation of health and social care in the United Kingdom and to the workforce that delivers care within these contexts. These highlight the need for occupational therapists to be flexible and adaptable in how and where they practice. Other changes that impact on occupational therapy practice might include advances in knowledge, social change, demographic change, technological change and changing social needs. If the profession wishes to have continued relevance to the delivery of health and social care that impacts on the occupational needs of society, then it will need to be transformational in its continued development.

Realising the vision through education

The purpose of occupational therapy education is to move the profession towards the realisation of the vision as set out in this document. In order to achieve this, two themes need to be integrated into educational programmes:

1 **The centrality of occupation in human life**
Occupation is essential both to individual health and wellbeing and to the health of communities and populations. Occupation is both the goal and the main tool of occupational therapists in their efforts to fulfil their professional purpose. Occupation must, therefore, be the core of the occupational therapy curriculum, into which all other subjects are integrated. The centrality of occupation in human life and in the occupational therapy curriculum must be made explicit.

2 **Transformation through occupation**
The purpose of occupational therapy is to transform individual lives, groups, communities and societies. The vehicle for this transformation is occupation. In order for students to experience the transformative potential of occupation, it must be demonstrated within the curriculum, so that learning itself becomes both an occupation and a vehicle for transformation.

For the profession to continue to move forwards, students must develop competence in three areas:

1 **Knowledge** including understanding of: the nature and importance of occupation to individuals, communities and populations; the relationship of occupation to health and wellbeing; the professional purpose of occupational therapy; and how occupational therapy works to improve health and wellbeing.

2 **Skill** including a broad range of: thinking and reasoning skills, interpersonal skills, occupational therapy process skills and skills in the use of activities as therapeutic media.

3 **Professionalism** including attitudes, values, beliefs, professional aspirations, professional identity, critical thinking and capability.

The overarching outcome of students' achievement of competence in these three areas will be their ability to articulate their professional purpose using the language of pragmatism. The curriculum must, therefore, be based on an appropriate and consistent use of professional language, since language is the vehicle through which occupational therapists articulate and defend their knowledge, skills and aptitudes. However, the curriculum must also take account of the need for occupational therapists to speak the language of a variety of employers and service users, in order to communicate effectively the dynamic nature of their services.

The theoretical basis of occupational therapy education must also be addressed. In spite of its pragmatic foundation, occupational therapy has commonly used a theoretical framework based in medicine to support its evolution and developing sense of its own credibility.

This difference between the profession's philosophical foundations and theoretical framework has not necessarily been made explicit in educational curricula. The tension between occupational therapy's professional values and knowledge base has sometimes led to confusion about: the legitimate purpose of the profession; the language used to represent key occupational therapy concepts; and what are seen as appropriate goals, processes and techniques for intervention.

The College of Occupational Therapists acknowledges the tensions that are known to exist, as noted above, yet recognises that appropriate medical knowledge is still necessary in order for graduates to be prepared for work within the predominantly medically-modelled ethos of the NHS. This curriculum guidance advocates inclusion of a balanced knowledge base that not only recognises the continuing needs of graduates who may be employed in the NHS, but also reflects the profession's maturing status. It is therefore important to also acknowledge the pragmatic aspects of occupational therapists' work and to develop better alignment between the knowledge base of the profession and its professional values. Graduates will thus be better prepared for future work both within and beyond the statutory sectors of health and social care.

The educational philosophy

It is a requirement of the College of Occupational Therapists that course teams within higher education institutions make explicit the educational philosophy that underpins the delivery of the curriculum. There should be a clear rationale that explains the links between the educational philosophy, the curriculum content and the way in which it is delivered. This guidance acknowledges that there are many educational approaches that may be used to support learning, including, for example:

- Problem-based, enquiry-based or task-based learning.
- Work-based learning.
- Experiential learning.
- Distance learning.
- Practice learning.
- Service learning.
- Independent learning.
- Online learning.

The above is not a definitive list. A variety of modes may be used within the programme. The main responsibility of the course team is to justify the approach(es) chosen and their congruence with occupational therapy philosophy.

The graduate profile

This curriculum guidance is a national guiding document for all occupational therapists in the UK and is the profession's view of what it wants its occupational therapy practitioners to embody. It is also an opportunity to take ownership of our professional capability and to articulate clearly how occupational therapy graduates can continue to contribute positively to the occupational needs of the population in support of people's health and wellbeing.

Graduates in occupational therapy will require a great number of skills, both profession-specific and generic. However, if it were possible to imagine what a future occupational therapist might be like, then aptitude descriptors such as confident, self-assured, considered risk-taker, culturally aware, grounded, politically astute, articulate and committed might be included. Such aptitudes may well be considered as requirements of the recruitment process but could be desirable equally as graduate outcomes. It is against this general background that the following graduate profile is set.

This profession-specific, graduate profile uses information adapted with permission from the following publication:

> Tuning Occupational Therapy Project Group (2008) *Reference points for the design and delivery of degree programmes in occupational therapy.* Bilbao: Publicaciones de la Universidad de Deusto.

Additional capabilities, or changes to existing competencies, are to contextualise the TUNING competencies within a UK context.

This profile is intended for use in curricula as a common statement of the profession's expected graduate competencies.

1. Knowledge and understanding of occupational therapy
The occupational therapy graduate is able to:

i Explain the philosophical and theoretical concepts underpinning occupational therapy, specifically the occupational nature of human beings and their performance of occupations.

ii Explain the relationship between occupational performance, health and wellbeing and the factors that facilitate or challenge participation in occupations, such as social difference, diversity and deprivation.

iii Synthesise theories of occupation and participation together with relevant knowledge from biological, medical, human, psychological, social, technological and occupational sciences.

iv Analyse the complexities of applying theories and research evidence related to occupation in the context of a changing society.

v Explain the impact of occupational dysfunction and deprivation on the occupational performance of individuals, families and communities, and the importance of restoring opportunities for participation in occupation.

vi Engage in rational and reasoned debate in relation to occupation and occupational therapy to critically evaluate and judge the impact of therapy on the service user.

2. Occupational therapy practice and professional reasoning
The occupational therapy graduate is able to:

i   Work in partnership with individuals and groups, using occupation in prevention, re/habilitation and treatment, in order to promote participation, health and wellbeing.

ii Take a person-centred approach in the assessment of the occupational needs of individuals, groups and communities and develop, implement and evaluate occupational therapy strategies to address them, through the selection, modification and application of theories, models of practice and approaches.

iii Utilise the therapeutic potential of occupation through the use of activity, occupational analysis and synthesis to enhance occupational function, taking account of the individual's rights, needs and preferences and ethical considerations.

iv Employ adaptive techniques in close collaboration with individuals and populations to facilitate accessible and adaptable environments in the promotion of occupational justice.

v   Collaborate with communities to promote and develop the health and wellbeing of their members through their participation in occupation.

vi Actively seek, critically evaluate and apply a range of information and evidence to ensure that occupational therapy practice is up to date and relevant to the client.

vii Critically appraise occupational therapy practice to ensure that the focus is on occupation and occupational performance and is attuned to the political and social context of the service.

viii Apply audit tools to determine occupational outcomes.

ix Use professional and ethical reasoning effectively throughout the occupational therapy episode.

3. Professional relationships and partnerships
The occupational therapy graduate is able to:

i   Work according to the principles of person-centred practice.

ii Build therapeutic relationships and partnerships as the foundation for occupational therapy intervention.

iii Establish and maintain collaborative partnerships, consult with and advise clients, carers, team members and other stakeholders on enabling occupation and participation in a wide range of contexts.

iv Collaborate with clients to advocate for the right to have their occupational needs met.

v   Appreciate and respect diversity, individual differences, cultural beliefs and customs and their influence on occupation and participation.

4. Professional autonomy and accountability

The occupational therapy graduate is able to:

i Prepare, maintain and review documentation related to their occupational therapy intervention.

ii Comply with professional standards, employer regulations and local/regional/ national/European policies and procedures.

iii Demonstrate acquisition of behaviours and skills congruent with the requirements of the current *College of Occupational Therapists' code of ethics and professional Conduct* (COT 2005, currently under review).

iv Demonstrate continuing lifelong learning to enhance occupational therapy practice.

v Demonstrate confidence in self-management, self-awareness and knowledge of own limitations as an occupational therapist.

5. Research and development in occupational therapy/science

The occupational therapy graduate is able to:

i Identify the need for research on issues related to occupation, occupational therapy and/or occupational science and formulate relevant research questions.

ii Search independently, critically examine, synthesise and utilise scientific literature and other information relevant to occupational therapy.

iii Understand, select and defend designs and methods appropriate to research in occupation and occupational therapy, including ethical considerations.

iv Interpret, analyse, synthesise and critique research findings relevant to occupational therapy.

v Contribute to the development of new knowledge of occupation and occupational therapy practice, particularly in relation to local and/or emerging health and social challenges.

vi Disseminate research findings in a variety of ways to a range of stakeholders.

6. Leadership and promotion of occupational therapy

The occupational therapy graduate is able to:

i Determine and prioritise occupational therapy services.

ii Understand and apply the principles of leadership and management to occupational therapy services, including the establishment of occupational therapy protocols.

iii Engage in a continuous process of evaluation and improvement of the quality of occupational therapy provision, involve users of services where appropriate and communicate results to others.

iv Take a proactive role in the development, improvement and promotion of occupational therapy.

v Proactively seek out and influence policies and legislation in health and social care locally, nationally and internationally that impact on occupational therapy services.

NB: This section is entitled 'Management and promotion of occupational therapy' in the original document.

In addition to the profession-specific competencies, there are a number of generic competencies that can be broadly summarised under the following headings:

- Communication skills: e.g. observation, listening, communication.
- Teamwork skills, including interprofessional working.
- Problem-setting and problem-solving skills.
- Educational skills in support of self-directed learning and learning of others.
- Business-mindedness, including risk assessment and cost/benefit analysis.
- Entrepreneurial, leadership and management skills.
- Marketing skills.
- Employability.
- Skills of reflection and self-evaluation.
- Research skills.
- Self-reliance and autonomy.
- Creativity and innovation.
- Coaching and mentoring skills.
- Ability to make independent judgements about complex issues.

Students should acquire these generic competencies at a level that is congruent with professional entry at honours level.

The competencies in these areas have been well documented by others. The College of Occupational Therapists has a keen interest in graduate professionals developing the skills above and recognises them as being complementary to those defined as specific to the profession. As such, the nature of their scope and depth is more appropriately defined by the higher education institution. In taking this approach, the College of Occupational Therapists has every confidence that education providers will be sensitive to the challenge of addressing interprofessional issues without compromising the quality or integrity of the professional programme(s).

Appendix

Current drivers impacting on the curriculum

A number of drivers currently impact on the occupational therapy curriculum. This document has been written to reflect those known drivers, but with some flexibility to accommodate an anticipated and, to some extent, an unanticipated future for the profession. The drivers (existing and new) that have been influential in the revision of the framework and that impact the four UK countries have been categorised in table A.1.

Table A.1: Current drivers impacting on the curriculum

Professional	Political
■ Ongoing focus on occupation.	■ The personalisation agenda.
■ Values and beliefs in occupation for health and wellbeing.	■ Increased expectations and purchasing power of service users.
■ Client-centred practice.	■ The significant changes in healthcare provision.
■ Evidence-informed/based practice and sharing of such evidence.	■ Increasing research capacity and funding streams to promote the development of research capacity at Masters and Doctoral levels.
■ Development of practice-driven research career pathways.	
■ Self-reliant practitioners.	■ Increased emphasis on health promotion.
■ Reflective and reflexive practitioners.	■ Emphasis on public health.
■ Flexible and adaptable practitioners.	■ Promotion of telecare and telehealth.
■ Interprofessional, multiprofessional and interagency working.	■ Strengthened political awareness and activity to develop occupational therapy practice.
■ Autonomy and accountability for professional work.	■ Expansion of practice to address the needs of individuals, groups, communities and populations.
■ Lifelong learning.	■ Community-based rehabilitation.
■ Clarity about the uniqueness of occupational therapy.	■ Government return-to-work agenda.
	■ Active ageing policies.
■ Development of the talents of occupational therapists in leadership, entrepreneurship, negotiation skills and business acumen.	■ Modernisation of allied health professions careers.
	■ Social inclusion; universal access to facilities.
■ Generation and use of outcome measures to recognise the impact of occupational therapy.	■ Widening participation in higher education.
	■ Marketing of the profession.
	■ Recovery model in mental health.
	■ Safeguarding.
	■ Better healthcare, wellbeing and quality of life for people with a learning disability.
National	**International**
■ Health Professions Council (HPC) *Standards of education and training* (2007).	■ Enhanced public health agenda.
■ HPC *Standards of proficiency* (2007).	■ Standards of the World Federation of Occupational Therapists (Hocking and Ness 2002).
■ HPC *Code of conduct* (2007).	
■ Increased community working.	■ International Classification of Function, Disability and Health (ICF).
■ Increased flexibility in working patterns across a seven day week.	■ The TUNING of curricula across Europe.
■ Increased work in the voluntary and independent sectors.	■ Internationalisation of curricula.
■ Changing demographics of the population.	■ Increased global mobility of occupational therapists.
■ Commissioning of competency-based packages.	

Other issues that influence the thinking around curriculum development

Knowledge base

The occupational therapy knowledge base (concepts, theories, models, frames of reference and approaches) is expanding to reflect increased political awareness and new areas of practice. Occupational science is recognised as informing much of the profession's practice. The integration of knowledge from many domains is required to deal with the increasing complexity of practice.

Emerging practice areas

The areas in which occupational therapists are employed are expanding. Areas that have proactively emerged and have been developed at the start of the 21st century continue to increase in number whilst new areas continue to evolve. This growth demonstrates that occupational therapists are recognised for their unique professional skills and occupational focus such that the profession can feel confident about its future in diverse settings. It is important therefore that future curricula prepare graduates for work with socially disaffected people.

Skills and attributes

The skills required by occupational therapists of the future will include many of those that have been traditionally expected and, in addition, will need to include those skills and aptitudes that enable occupational therapists to take a business-minded approach to their practice. Thus, the skills required by the occupational therapist of the future would include those that reflect the current and developing areas of practice. The specific capabilities are identified in the graduate profile (see pages 10–13).

The educational context

It is important to recognise that issues affecting the educational context need to be considered by Higher Education Institutions in the recruitment and retention of students and in learning, teaching and assessment strategies. These currently include:

- Student demographics.
- Social inclusion.
- Widening participation.
- Recruitment of students who understand their future role.
- Accommodation of students with specific needs.
- Flexible learning patterns.
- Learning from service users.
- Interprofessional learning.
- Use of technology for learning and professional development.
- Lifelong learning.
- Learning for employability.
- Concept of graduateness.

Bibliography and references

Audi R ed (1999) *The Cambridge dictionary of philosophy.* 2nd ed. Cambridge: Cambridge University Press.

Butterfield J ed (2003) *Collins English Dictionary: complete and unabridged.* 6th ed. Glasgow: Harper Collins.

College of Occupational Therapists (2008) *College of Occupational Therapists pre-registration education standards.* London: COT.

College of Occupational Therapists (2005) *College of Occupational Therapists code of ethics and professional conduct.* London: COT.

Creek J (2003) *Occupational therapy defined as a complex intervention.* London: College of Occupational Therapists.

Health Professions Council (2007a) *Code of conduct.* London: HPC.

Health Professions Council (2007b) *Standards of education and training.* London: HPC.

Health Professions Council (2007c) *Standards of proficiency: occupational therapists.* London: HPC.

Hocking C and Ness N E (2002) *Revised minimum standards for the education of occupational therapists.* Sidney: World Federation of Occupational Therapists.

Hooper B, Wood W (2002) Pragmatism and structuralism in occupational therapy: the long conversation. *American Journal of Occupational Therapy, 56(1),* 40–50.

Short E (1985) The concept of competence: its use and misuse in education. *Journal of Teacher Education, 36(2),* 2–6.

Trumble W R, Stevenson A (2002) *Shorter Oxford English Dictionary.* 5th ed. Oxford: Oxford University Press.

Tuning Occupational Therapy Project Group (2008) *Reference points for the design and delivery of degree programmes in occupational therapy.* Bilbao: Publicaciones de la Universidad de Deusto.

Vickers A (2007) Patterns of transformative learning. *Widening Participation and Lifelong Learning, 9(3),* 38–46.

Wilcock A A (2006) *An occupational perspective of health.* 2nd ed. Thorofare, New Jersey: Slack.